Conte

Interstitial Cystitis Diet Cookbook

INTRODUCTION

Vegetables are not only rich in nutrients and antioxidants, but most of them are safe on an interstitial cystitis diet. Vegetables are also versatile elements of a healthy diet. Eat them raw or cooked, or throw them in a blender to add powerful nutrients to your smoothies. Frozen vegetables are just as healthy as fresh, so fill your freezer with frozen broccoli, Brussels sprouts, peas, and corn. Carrots, celery, cucumbers, potatoes, squash, and greens are inexpensive staples that can help you design a menu full of colorful goodness. By keeping these comfort food staples on hand, you can quickly throw together a stir-fry or soup! Portion size is also important when you are considering troublesome foods like tomatoes. You just may be able to have one slice of tomato on a sandwich, but a cup of tomato pasta sauce is too much.

Vegetables, Salads, and Soups List

Note: Foods labeled with a plus sign (+) may be especially soothing during an IC flare according to patient reports.

Bladder Friendly

Asparagus

Avocado

Beans – black eyed peas, garbanzo, lentils, pinto, white, most dried beans

Beets

Bell peppers – yellow, orange, red

Broccoli

Brussels sprouts

Cabbage

Carrots+

Cauliflower

Celery

Chives

Corn+

Cucumber

Eggplant

Green beans

Greens – collard greens, kale, mustard greens, okra, Swiss chard, spinach, bok choy

Lettuce & most salad greens

Mushrooms

Olives – black

Parsley

Peas – green+, snow peas, split peas

Potatoes+– white, yams

Pumpkin

Radishes

Rhubarb

Rutabaga

Homemade soup & stock – from okay meats and vegetables

Squash+ – summer, winter, zucchini

Turnips

Try It

beans – fava, kidney beans, lima beans, black beans

bell peppers – green

olives – green

greens – chicory, dandelion greens, purslane, turnip greens

leeks (cooked)

Onions – white, red, cooked bulb onion, raw green

Soups – canned, low sodium, organic soups (without problem ingredients)

tomatoes – homegrown, low acid

Watercress

Bouillon – cubes, powder

Chili peppers

kimchi

onions – raw bulb onions

Pickles

sauerkraut

soup – most canned, boxed

soy beans – edamame, roasted

tomato – tomato sauces, tomato juice

tofu

No time for breakfast? No IC appropriate or convenient choices? This recipe practically makes itself with just a bit of effort the night before. So make mornings less chaotic and join the "overnight oats" bandwagon without irritating your IC.

RECIPES

IC Overnight Apple and Almond Oats

Yields: 1 serving Prep time: 5 minutes

small jelly jar and lid or 8 oz canning jar and lid

Ingredients

1/2 cup old fashioned oats (or steel cut or gluten free if needed)

1/2 cup lowfat milk

1/3 cup plain lowfat yogurt

1/2 teaspoon cinnamon (if tolerated)

Pinch of salt

1/2 cup chopped, fresh apple slices with peel

Tablepoon sliced almonds

1/2 tablespoon honey

Directions

In a small resealable jar combine oats, milk, yogurt, cinnamon and salt. Seal jar with a lid and shake well. Refrigerate overnight. Top with fruit and honey and eat.

15 IC Friendly Grocery Items To Have On Hand

Everyone wants an IC grocery shopping list. Well, I couldn't come up with one that would satisfy everyone, but I do have these recommendations for the top 15 healthiest choices.

FRIDGE:

Eggs – Try Omega-3 eggs (like Eggland's Best) for anti-inflammatory properties, or any for a complete protein source and quick meals

Baby spinach/greens – Nature's nutrient power-house (vitamin A, C, Calcium, fiber, folate, potassium and anti-oxidants) toss in pasta or soup or "hide" by blenderizing into sauces or smoothies

Colored Sweet Bell Peppers – Not the green or hot ones, twice as much vitamin C as an orange and a terrific tomato substitute – easy to oven roast to really bring out the flavor

Apples – Gala and Fuji are most IC friendly, only 80 calories, full of fiber and sweet. Other types (not Granny Smith) are "try-it"s. Topping for oatmeal and a snack mate for peanut butter

Greek Yogurt – It may be a "try-it" item, but so full of calcium, protein, magnesium, probiotics and vitamin D. Organic types may have less sugar and fewer preservatives. Skip artificially sweetened and those flavored with "avoid" fruits and flavors

FROZEN:

Blueberries – Frozen, fresh or dried – a super source of vitamin C, fiber and anti-oxidants – the best cranberry substitute. Raspberries blackberries and cherries are "try-it" options

90% lean turkey or chicken – check labels and avoid those with "added broth", flavorings and preservatives. High in protein, iron, zinc and fewer calories than beef

Frozen veggies – Frozen can retain more nutrients than "fresh" depending how long it's been sitting at the store or traveling. Avoid added sauces and season with IC friendly herbs

Frozen Shrimp – low-cal, high protein – so easy for quick dinners or an appetizer. Excellent with basil pesto

PANTRY:

Pouch "tuna style" salmon or light tuna – a major source of Omega 3's, a low-cal protein and at times the only appetizing seafood available. A patty recipe on the label was IC friendly minus the Worcestershire sauce

Nuts – Almonds, peanuts and cashews – not just for snacking – filling and chock full of anti-inflammatory oils, vegetarian, gluten-free, fiber, iron, vitamin E and a good source of protein. If calories are a concern – limit to 20-30 per serving

Nut Butters – Don't be afraid of the price. Compared to meat it's a cheap protein alternative and an amazing apple, celery topper

Canned (or frozen) lentils, chick peas and white beasns – Tons of fiber, protein and healthy carbs – another cheap IC meat sub. Rinse, season with garlic, salt and pepper, olive oil and basil then toss with roasted red peppers and pasta or salad – no cooking!

Oats – Learn to love it, an IC lifesaver! Bladder-soothing, high fiber and all natural. Make ahead and refrigerate to save time

Olive Oil – Heart healthy, anti-inflammatory and a few teaspoons with herbs adds lots of flavor and not too many calories.

IC Butternut Squash and Kale Lasagna

Having a big gathering at your place? Here is a recipe that will satisfy large crowds and keep your IC happy.

Tomato based sauce can be offered on the side or added to the layers in a second pan for those without IC.

Serves 6-8

Pre-heat oven to 400 degrees and grease or spray a 9 by 13 inch baking dish

Ingredients

2 Tbsp olive oil

1 medium butternut squash, peeled and cut into small cubes

1 Tbsp brown sugar

Sea salt and fresh ground black pepper

3 cloves fresh garlic, peeled and diced

1/4 tsp nutmeg (if tolerated although in this quantity, may not be a problem)

2 tsps fresh thyme, chopped

1 bunch kale, washed, stems removed and chopped or a large container of baby spinach washed, stems removed and chopped

(About 4 cups)

1 pound low-fat ricotta cheese

Another 1/2 tsp nutmeg

6 fresh sage sprigs, chopped and 2 more for topping

Mozzarella cheese, low-fat or regular, shredded to make 1/2 cup plus some to sprinkle on top if desired

1 cup fresh pecorino cheese, grated (or fresh grated parmesan) plus 2-3 Tbsp to sprinkle on top

1/3 cup low-fat milk

1 pound no-boil lasagna noodles, whole wheat (or 1 pound pasta)

2 Tbsp pumpkin seeds to sprinkle on top

Directions

Preheat oven to 400 degrees. Heat olive oil in a large skillet over medium heat. Add butternut squash and sprinkle with brown sugar and season with sea salt and fresh ground pepper. Cook for 10-15 minutes stirring frequently to avoid burning until browned. Add garlic, nutmeg, and thyme, cook 5 minutes more.

Remove from heat and add kale, cover and let sit 10 minutes until kale wilts.

In a large bowl mix ricotta cheese with remaining 1/2 tsp nutmeg, sage, mozzarella cheese, pecorino or parmesan cheese and milk. Season with salt and pepper.

Heavily spray or butter a 9 by 13 baking dish and layer with 1/3 of the lasagna noodles. Add 1/3 of the kale/squash mixture layered over the noodles. Add 1/3 of the cheese mixture and drizzle with a little olive oil.

Repeat the layering 2 more times or until all is used. Drizzle a little olive oil over top. Sprinkle with pecorino or parmesan and sage leaves as the top layer. If you like a browned, crunchy top, add a final topping of mozzarella after initial baking and bake 10 more minutes or until mozzarella is browned.

Cover with foil sprayed with cooking spray and refrigerate up to 3 days. Or bake immediately at 400 degrees for 35-45 minutes and uncovered 10 more if topping with mozzarella. If you are baking after refrigeration, add 15-20 minutes to baking time.

Sprinkle with pumpkin seeds (or pine nuts) and serve.

IC FRIENDLY CREAMY CHICKEN AND VEGETABLES

Ingredients

2 cups of cooked, chunked chicken

1 15-oz. can pure, organic chicken or vegetable broth (or stock from home-cooked chicken)

10 fresh mushrooms, sliced

1/4 cup chopped sweet onion (if tolerated) or substitute 2 teaspoons IC Friendly fresh, minced garlic

1/4 teaspoon dried or 1 tablespoon fresh oregano

1/8 teaspoon fresh, ground pepper

1 cup frozen green peas

1 cup frozen mixed veggies (broccoli cuts, carrots, cauliflower florets, etc.)

2 tablespoons cornstarch

2 – 4 tablespoons grated Parmesan cheese (if tolerated) or shredded mozzarella

Directions

Place all ingredients except chicken broth, cornstarch and grated cheese in a large saucepan. Mix together. Reserve 1/2 cup broth. Add remaining broth to the pan. Bring the mixture to a boil and simmer until vegetables are cooked.

Mix reserved broth, cornstarch and cheese. Stir the mixture into the other ingredients and boil for one minute to thicken. Serve over a favorite rice, pasta or phyllo or pie crust baked in muffin cups. Serves 4 – 6.

WHITE CHOCOLATE CHUNK COOKIES IC RECIPE

Ingredients

1 cup sugar

1 cup brown sugar

1 cup softened butter

1/2 cup canola oil

1 egg, beaten

1 teaspoon vanilla extract

1 tablespoon milk

3 1/2 cups flour

1 teaspoon baking soda

1 teaspoon cream of tartar

1 teaspoon salt

1 cup white "chocolate", organic chips or chunks (find those with the fewest ingredients to avoid preservatives if bothersome) peanut butter or butterscotch chips are also good (if tolerated) or substitute a cup of IC friendly carob chips

1 cup brown or golden raisins (if tolerated) or substitute 1/2 cup IC friendly chopped almonds or cashews

Directions

Beat together sugars, butter, vegetable oil, egg, vanilla and milk. Mix in flour, baking soda, cream of tartar and salt. Stir in white chocolate chips & raisins. Drop onto a greased or parchment papered cookie sheet and bake at 350 degrees for about 13 minutes. Tops should be light brown. Makes 4 – 5 dozen.

Leftover Turkey Pot pies for IC diet

Turkey pot pie

Here is a recipe from Parade Magazine that is adaptable to the IC diet.

Serves 4 Pre-heat oven to 375 degrees and line a rimmed baking sheet with foil

Ingredients:

4 T butter

1 T diced garlic

2 medium carrots, peeled and thinly sliced

1 stick of celery, thinly sliced

Salt and pepper

4 T flour

2 1/2 cups turkey, chicken or vegetable broth (low sodium, organic)

1/4 cup heavy cream or milk

3/4 tsp dried or 2 tsp fresh thyme, chopped

1 1/2 cups cooked, shredded skinless turkey or chicken meat (organic, broth-free or preservative free)

1/2 cup peas

2 T chopped fresh parsley

1 sheet frozen puff pastry, thawed (some contain citric acid low on the ingredient list – a try-it item)

1 large egg

Preparation:

Warm butter in a large saucepan on low heat. Add garlic, carrot and celery, sprinkle with salt and pepper and cook, stirring occasionally until tender 10 min.

Sprinkle with flour and cook 3 min, stirring constantly. Pour in broth and cream/milk. Stir in thyme. Bring to a simmer over medium heat. Reduce heat and gently simmer 10 min until thick and stir to prevent sticking.

Remove from heat. Stir in chicken or turkey, peas and parsley. Divide into 4 8 ounce ramekins. Place on rimmed, foil-covered baking sheet.

Place puff pastry on lightly floured surface. Slice into 4 inch squares and place over ramekins.

Whisk egg and 1 T water in a small bowl. Brush pastry tops with egg mixture.

Bake until golden and bubbly about 35 minutes in 375 degree oven. Let stand 5 min then serve.

IC Diet Herbed Chicken with Asparagus

Spring!? Where is it? Well, at least the spring asparagus is available and IC Friendly, too! Enjoy!

HERBED CHICKEN WITH ASPARAGUS

Ingredients

1/4 cup flour

2 tablespoons grated Parmesan cheese (if tolerated or try mozzarella)

1/2 teaspoon fresh, diced garlic (or powder)

1/4 teaspoon black pepper

1 pound thin-sliced boneless skinless chicken breasts (without added broth if it is irritating)

1 tablespoon olive oil

1 1/2 cups pure chicken stock (cook a chicken or try canned organic for the least irritating ingredients)

1 teaspoon basil

1 teaspoon oregano

1 pound asparagus, trimmed and cut into 1-inch pieces

Instructions

In a shallow dish, mix flour, cheese, garlic and pepper. Reserve 2 tablespoons. Moisten chicken lightly with water. Coat evenly with remaining flour mixture.

In a large nonstick skillet, heat oil on medium heat. Add half of the chicken pieces; cook 3 minutes per side, or until golden brown. Repeat with remaining chicken, adding additional oil, if necessary. Remove chicken from skillet; keep warm.

In medium bowl, mix stock, basil, oregano and reserved flour mixture until well blended. Add to skillet along with asparagus.

Bring to boil. Reduce heat to low; simmer 3-5 minutes, or until sauce is slightly thickened, stirring frequently. Return chicken to skillet and cook until heated through. Serves 4.

IC WHITE BEAN CHICKEN CHILI

One of our special IC patients is a valuable resource for recipes that are appropriate for IC. Here is her healthy chili choice that will warm you up without irritating your bladder. The recipe can be modified as indicated for vegetarian chili. Perfect for Fall!!

Ingredients

1 tablespoon olive oil

1 cup chopped sweet onion (if tolerated)

1 cup chopped celery

2 sweet bell peppers cored and chopped (red, yellow or orange or green if tolerated)

1 pound ground lean chicken or turkey with no preservatives (for vegetarian chili substitute 1 can of beans and 1 cup of corn)

It is also possible to use 2 cups grilled chicken breast or turkey tenderloin instead of ground

1 tablespoon minced garlic

1 tablespoon all-purpose flour

1 teaspoon ground cumin (if tolerated or substitute dried basil)

1 teaspoon dried oregano

2 cups chicken or vegetable broth low-sodium or with no preservatives

2 15 ounce cans white beans drained and rinsed (mash one can of beans for thicker chili)

1/2 cup low-fat sour cream or plain yogurt (if tolerated)

Salt and pepper to taste

Shredded mild cheddar cheese for topping and/or can chopped mild green chilis if tolerated

In a large pot over medium heat warm the oil. Add chopped veggies and sautee for 5 min. Add chicken or turkey and cook through at least 5 minutes. Omit for vegetarian chili.

Add the garlic, flour, cumin (or basil) and oregano. Cook, stirring over low heat 2 minutes. Add the broth while stirring. Increase heat and bring to a boil stirring occasionally. Reduce heat to simmering and cook 10 minutes longer.

Add the beans and simmer another 10 minutes. Mash 1 can of the beans for thicker chili. Add a third can of beans and corn for vegetarian chili.

Stir in sour cream or yogurt. Season with salt and pepper.

Ladle into bowls and top with shredded cheddar and green chilis. May be served over rice, quinoa or other cooked grains.

Add a warm piece of corn bread for a more hearty meal. Serves about 6.

Quick Breakfast Pizza for IC diets

Breakfast, lunch, dinner or snack – something everyone can enjoy

IC PIZZA – EGGS, CHEESE and SAUSAGE

For the crust:

1 3/4 cups Bisquick (all IC friendly except for a small amount of "try it" list soybean oil)

* A homemade, soybean oil-free "Bisquick" recipe follows

** or substitute a homemade 12″ pizza crust recipe – prepared crusts may contain irritating ingredients

1/4 cup grated Parmesan cheese (if tolerated)

1/2 teaspoon onion powder (if tolerated) or substitute garlic powder

1/3 cup water

2 tablespoons olive oil

For the filling:

3 large eggs

1 cup pure sour cream (Daisy brand is good but is a "try it" ingredient)

1 1/2 teaspoons fresh dill or 1/2 teaspoon dried dill or substitute basil if desired

1/4 teaspoon salt

1 cup shredded mozzarella or mild cheddar cheese

1/3 cup each of sweet onion (if tolerated) and fresh or roasted red bell pepper, chopped or sliced

1 crushed garlic bulb section (about 1 teaspoon minced) optional

8 ounces sliced sweet Italian chicken sausage links (Al Fresco brand available at Meijer is I.C. friendly) or substitute grilled, shredded fresh chicken breast

To make the crust:

Heat oven to 425 degrees. Coat a 12-inch pizza pan with non-stick cooking spray. Combine Bisquick, Parmesan cheese and onion powder in medium bowl, stirring until blended. Stir in water and olive oil until dough forms. Press dough onto bottom of prepared pan to form a crust, building up outside edge to form a rim. Bake for 7 minutes.

For the filling:

Whisk eggs, sour cream, dill and salt in medium bowl. Stir in cheese, onion, bell pepper and/or garlic. Pour over hot crust, spreading evenly. Place sliced sausage or chicken over egg mixture. Reduce oven to 350 degrees. Bake 20-25 minutes until egg mixture is set in center. Cool 5 minutes before cutting. Good for breakfast, lunch or dinner!

* Homemade Bisquick mix substitution recipe: Mix in a large bowl – 2 cups flour, 3 teaspoons baking powder, 1 teaspoon salt, and 2 tablespoons butter. Cut butter into flour with a fork or a whisk until mixture resembles fine crumbs. Store in an airtight container in a cool, dry place up to 2 months.

Many other vegetables can be added or substituted such as spinach leaves, mushrooms, black olives, steamed broccoli or asparagus.

IC CREAMY CHICKEN AND VEGETABLES AND IC WHITE CHOCOLATE CHUNK COOKIES

Celebrate the New Year with 2 IC-safe recipes that can be shared with non-IC friends. Great ideas for a winter pot-luck!!

Ingredients

2 cups of cooked, chunked chicken

1 15-oz. can pure, organic chicken or vegetable broth (or stock from home-cooked chicken)

10 fresh mushrooms, sliced

1/4 cup chopped sweet onion (if tolerated) or substitute 2 teaspoons IC Friendly fresh, minced garlic

1/4 teaspoon dried or 1 tablespoon fresh oregano

1/8 teaspoon fresh, ground pepper

1 cup frozen green peas

1 cup frozen mixed veggies (broccoli cuts, carrots, cauliflower florets, etc.)

2 tablespoons cornstarch

2 – 4 tablespoons grated Parmesan cheese (if tolerated) or shredded mozzarella

Instructions

Place all ingredients except chicken broth, cornstarch and grated cheese in a large saucepan. Mix together. Reserve 1/2 cup broth. Add remaining broth to the pan. Bring the mixture to a boil and simmer until vegetables are cooked. Mix reserved broth, cornstarch and cheese. Stir the mixture into the other ingredients and boil for one minute to thicken. Serve over a favorite rice, pasta or phyllo or pie crust baked in muffin cups. Serves 4 – 6.

WHITE CHOCOLATE CHUNK COOKIES IC RECIPE

Ingredients

1 cup sugar

1 cup brown sugar

1 cup softened butter

1/2 cup canola oil

1 egg, beaten

1 teaspoon vanilla extract

1 tablespoon milk

3 1/2 cups flour

1 teaspoon baking soda

1 teaspoon cream of tartar

1 teaspoon salt

1 cup white "chocolate", organic chips or chunks (find those with the fewest ingredients to avoid preservatives if bothersome) peanut butter or butterscotch

chips are also good (if tolerated) or substitute a cup of IC friendly carob chips

1 cup brown or golden raisins (if tolerated) or substitute 1/2 cup IC friendly chopped almonds or cashews

Instructions

Beat together sugars, butter, vegetable oil, egg, vanilla and milk. Mix in flour, baking soda, cream of tartar and salt. Stir in white chocolate chips & raisins. Drop onto a greased or parchment papered cookie sheet and bake at 350 degrees for about 13 minutes. Tops should be light brown. Makes 4 – 5 dozen.

Spinach and Cheese Pizza – IC Friendly

Prep Time: 5 minutes

Cook Time: 20 minutes

Yield: Makes: 4 servings (serving size: 2 slices)

Ingredients

All-purpose flour and cornmeal

1 pound whole-wheat pizza dough, room temperature

1 1/2 tablespoons olive oil

1 jumbo onion, halved and thinly sliced (if tolerated) or substitute cloves roasted sliced garlic

1/8 teaspoon salt

1/8 teaspoon pepper (if tolerated)

10 ounce fresh chopped spinach

3 tablespoons feta cheese

Directions

1. Place an oven rack on lowest position and preheat to 500°F.

2. On a lightly floured surface, roll dough into a 14-inch round. Generously sprinkle a baking sheet with cornmeal. Place dough on sheet. Bake until crisp, about 12 minutes.

3. Heat oil in a nonstick skillet on medium-high. Add onion (or garlic), salt and pepper (if tolerated). Cook, stirring, until golden. Add 1/4 cup water, cover and cook on low until soft. Stir in spinach; spoon on crust, leaving a 1/2-inch border. Crumble cheese on top.

4. Bake for 5 minutes. Cut into 8 slices. Serve.

IC Friendly Spring Greens – Ideas and Recipes

With Spring finally here vary your daily salad and vegetable servings with these raw and cooked 10 great arugula ideas. These recipes will work with any tender spring green; try spinach, watercress, mesclun, dandelion, or young mustard greens.

Eat It Raw:

Use about 9 oz (8 cups) arugula for each salad and add the other ingredients to taste. Dress lightly with herb-infused olive oil, lemon zest (if tolerated), and salt and pepper (if tolerated), or use your favorite IC friendly homemade dressing.

1. Italian

Arugula, sliced radicchio, Parmesan cheese shavings (if tolerated) or fresh sliced mozzarella, quartered artichoke hearts, pitted black olives

2. Summer

Arugula, diced sweet red bell pepper, fresh corn kernels, fresh basil

3. Steakhouse

Arugula, sliced steak, cucumber, chopped scallions, crisp bacon (if tolerated)

4. Sweet and Salty

Arugula, diced fresh pears, crumbled feta cheese, toasted, lightly salted cashews

5. California

Arugula, crumbled Feta, toasted candied almonds, dried or fresh blueberries

Try It Cooked:

1. Pesto

Puree 2 garlic cloves, 2 cups packed arugula, ½ cup olive oil, and ¼ cup cashews or pinenuts. Add 1 Tbsp lemon zest (if tolerated); season with salt and pepper. Serve on grilled fish or chicken.

2. Pilaf

Sauté 1 diced onion (if tolerated) or garlic in 2 Tbsp canola oil in a pot. Add 1½ cups rice, 2½ cups water, and salt to taste. Bring to a simmer. Stir in ¼ cup raisin (if tolerated)s and ¼ cup -slivered almonds. When rice is tender, stir in 2 cups packed a rugula.

3. Sandwich

Layer slices of ripe peach (if tolerated) or fresh sliced fuji apples, thin slices of Gruyère cheese, and a handful of arugula between 2 slices of whole wheat bread. Bake until cheese melts.

4. Pasta

Combine ¾ lb cooked whole wheat spaghetti, 1/2 cup steamed mushrooms, 1/2 cup steamed carrots, with 2 cups packed arugula, ¼ cup chopped parsley, 3 Tbsp pine nuts, 1 Tbsp olive oil, and salt and pepper to taste. Warm.

5. Pizza

Top a whole wheat pizza crust with -basil pesto, a handful of arugula, sautéed broccoli, and shredded mozzarella. Bake at 425°F until cheese melts.

Tuna and White Bean Bruschetta for IC

Ingredients

Sliced whole-grain or white french bread, toasted and buttered

1/2 to 1 teaspoon minced garlic

15-ounce can white beans, drained and rinsed

6 tablespoons extra-virgin olive oil

Two 5-ounce cans pure light tuna packed in water, drained and flaked (check for one without soybean oil)

3/4 cup finely chopped celery

1/2 cup finely chopped sweet onion (if tolerated)

3/4 cup pitted and chopped natural black olives packed in water (yes, these are IC friendly!)

Zest of 1 lemon (only if tolerated, this a "try it" item)

1 tablespoon fresh or dried oregano or basil

2 cups baby arugula or other small greens like fresh spinach

Instructions

Toast and butter bread; set aside.

In a large bowl use a potato masher or fork to mash the beans.

Add the olive oil, tuna, celery, onion, olives, lemon zest, oregano, minced garlic and greens.

Mix gently, season with salt and pepper. Spread the mixture on top of the sliced bread.

Salad with Honey-Drizzled Pears – IC Diet Friendly

Prep time: 20 minutes

Total Time: 20 minutes

Salad with honey-drizzled pears and goat cheese rounds. Shown with optional peaches if tolerated.

Ingredients:

¼ cup (s) almonds, toasted, finely chopped

½ tsp kosher salt, divided

4 oz goat cheese

4 oz OR 6 cups salad greens – arugula or spinach, any other

1 tbsp olive oil

1 medium lemon – zest only

4 medium pears, fresh (ripe but firm) or canned

2 tbsp honey

Ground black pepper (optional)

*substitutions: peaches if tolerated

Instructions:

1. Place almonds in shallow dish. Season with ¼ tsp salt and optional pepper. Roll goat cheese log in pecans to coat. Refrigerate the log until firm, if necessary, then cut into 8 rounds.

2. Place greens into medium bowl. Add oil and lemon zest and toss to coat. Season with remaining ¼ tsp salt and optional pepper.

3. Divide the salad greens among 4 shallow bowls. Nestle 2 pear halves into each portion or greens, top each half with a round of almond crusted goat cheese and drizzle each salad with honey.

Basil Blueberry Non-Vinaigrette Salad Dressing

Ingredients

1 c. frozen blueberries, partially thawed

1/2 c. organic, pure blueberry juice

1/2 c. olive oil

1 t. lemon zest

1/2 t. sugar

2 t. finely chopped fresh basil (may substitute thyme)

Pinch salt

Pinch white pepper as tolerated to taste

Instructions

Place all ingredients in blender. Blend using one-second "pulses," checking consistency after every couple of pulses.

May also be made without using frozen berries. Simply increase juice to 1 cup.

Homemade and Healthy Ranch Salad Dressing

Ingredients

1 c. fat - free plain yogurt (try organic Greek yogurt!)

1/2 c. low - fat cottage cheese

1/2 t. lemon zest

1 t. dill

2 t. parsley

1/4 t. minced garlic

Pinch onion powder

Pinch sugar

Salt and pepper to taste, if tolerated

Instructions

Blend all ingredients in blender or food processor until smooth. Store in refrigerator for up to one week past "sell - by" dates on yogurt and cottage cheese.

9 Things to do with canned pumpkin if you have IC:

Stir a spoonful into plain (or vanilla) yogurt and a bit of honey (cinnamon if tolerated)

Add a dollop to a morning yogurt smoothie

Makes a flavorful and nutritious addition to cheesecake recipes many of which can be made low fat and without the potentially IC irritating graham cracker or ginger snap crust

Add about 1/3 cup to pancake batter making 8-10 pancakes. Add chopped apples and top with a little pure maple syrup

Makes a delectable IC friendly sauce for cheese ravioli (for those handy in the kitchen, making pumpkin-stuffed ravioli is another option)

A unique addition to risotto recipes in place of butternut squash

Delicious and smooth as a savory fall soup

Just stir a tsp or two into low fat cream cheese and a bit of honey for a new twist on breakfast bagels or English muffins

From a 1980's copy of Country Living Magazine: Beef and Pumpkin Stew

A spoonful of canned pumpkin is an ideal addition to pet food to help older dogs with sensitive stomachs or cats prone to hairballs by keeping them "regular". Dogs love it, not sure about cats

IC Friendly Appetizers: Holiday Dips

PUMPKIN-MAPLE DIP

In a food processor, combine a 4-oz. package (not tub) room temperature cream cheese, 1/2 cup canned pumpkin puree, 1/4 cup plain Greek yogurt, 3 tablespoons maple syrup, 2 tablespoons peanut butter, 1/2 teaspoon ground cinnamon (if tolerated) and a pinch of salt. Process until smooth. Place in serving bowl.

Serve with sliced Gala or Fuji apples, Ace brand whole wheat bread (no preservatives) or graham crackers (if tolerated). Makes 2 cups.

CARAMELIZED ONION AND WHITE BEAN DIP

In a large skillet, warm 2 tablespoons olive oil over low heat. Add 2 large thinly sliced sweet onions (cooking onions sometimes makes them more tolerable); sprinkle with salt and pepper and cook, stirring occasionally, until deeply browned, about 40 minutes. If onions start to burn, add a little water and stir. Remove from heat and cool slightly. Set aside 1 tablespoon onions for garnish. Place remainder in a food processor with 1 14-oz. can drained and rinsed white beans, 1/4 cup sour cream or plain Greek yogurt and 2-3 tablespoons olive oil. Puree until smooth. Salt and pepper to taste. Place into serving bowl and top with reserved onions.

Serve with potato chips (check ingredients: IC friendly chips contain potatoes, vegetable oil, no soybean oil and salt) sliced veggies like IC friendly carrots, celery, broccoli, cauliflower and our favorite, red, orange and yellow sweet bell peppers (green if tolerated), or a preservative free whole wheat pita or flat bread. Makes about 2 cups.

If you don't have a food processor, a blender or hand mixer works.

Quinoa and Vegetable Pilaf – IC Friendly

Ingredients:

1 3/4 c organic low-sodium broth if tolerated or homemade stock from cooked whole chicken

1 cup quinoa rinsed and drained *

2 Tbsp olive oil

2 tsp or more minced garlic

2 cups diced red and yellow bell pepper and/or carrots

1 cup chopped asparagus or green beans

1 cup diced zucchini and/or yellow summer squash

1/4 tsp sea salt

1/4 tsp black pepper if tolerated

2 tsp lemon zest if tolerated

1/2 c crumbled feta cheese

1 Tbsp chopped, fresh parsley or basil

Instructions:

In a saucepan bring broth to a boil. Add quinoa, cover and reduce heat to simmering. Cook quinoa until tender, about 15 minutes, stirring occasionally.

Remove from heat, fluff with a fork. Heat oil in a large skillet over medium heat. Add garlic and vegetables. Season with salt and pepper if tolerated.

Saute until tender, 7-8 minutes. Add quinoa, lemon zest and feta. Spoon into serving dishes and sprinkle with parsley or basil.

* A quick substitute for quinoa is microwaveable Minute Rice Multi-Grain Medley 4 ready-to-serve cups (contains brown rice, wheat, quinoa, rye and barley) added to broth and heated (not boiled). Drain unabsorbed, excess broth before adding to vegetables if necessary. Add cooked black lentils or rinsed canned garbanzo beans when adding vegetables for antioxidants, protein and fiber.

Nutrition: 280 calories, 35 gm carb, 11 gm protein, 10 gm fat, 510 mg sodium and 5 gm fiber per 1 of 4 servings.

Crustless Zucchini Pie – IC friendly

Even though it doesn't LOOK like Spring – Let's celebrate!!

Zucchini is great in many IC dishes, but this takes the cake – I mean pie.

Ingredients

4 cups zucchini, thin-sliced or grated (don't peel it)

1 cup sliced sweet onion if tolerated, or substitute 1/4 cup diced, IC friendly fresh chives)

1/2 cup butter or margarine

2 teaspoons parsley flakes or 1-2 tablespoon fresh chopped

1/2 teaspoon salt

1/2 teaspoon pepper

1/4 teaspoon garlic powder or 1 – 2 cloves diced fresh

1/4 teaspoon dried basil or 2 teaspoons diced fresh

1/4 teaspoon dried oregano or 2 teaspoons diced fresh

2 eggs

12 ounces Shredded mozzarella cheese

Instructions

Place zucchini, onion & butter in fry pan. Cook ten minutes, until soft. Add parsley flakes, salt, pepper, garlic powder, basil, oregano; stir. Turn off heat.

Beat eggs in bowl; add cheese.

Pour zucchini mixture into greased pie plate. Cover with cheese mixture. Bake at 350 degrees for 20 minutes. Good hot or cold.

PS: This recipe can be modified many ways. Substitute broccoli or spinach or combine all with mushrooms for a vegetable pie. Try a little shredded cheddar cheese. Don't forget a decorative yet edible garnish like fresh basil leaves, or sliced black olives or for a pop of color add sliced strips of sweet red bell pepper before baking. Individual tart pans can be used as well.

IC Pasta Sauce

3 bell peppers, sliced (red, yellow, orange)

1/2 cup sweet onion, sliced (if tolerated or 2 teaspoons diced garlic)

2 tablespoons olive oil

1 can (18.8 oz.) Campbell's Home Style or Natural Butternut Squash Bisque Soup (if you are especially sensitive, substitute a lower sodium version like Imagine brand Light in Sodium Creamy Butternut Squash soup in a 32 ounce shelf stable box. Use a little more than half.)

Instructions

In large frying pan, saute vegetables for 15 minutes until tender. Place cooked vegetables into blender; add soup. Blend until desired consistency is reached. Season with salt, pepper, garlic powder, Italian herbs, etc. to taste. Serve over cooked white, whole wheat or tri-color pasta or ravioli. Makes 4 cups. Freeze any extra sauce.

Garnsh with fresh basil or sage and a sprinkle of grated mozzarella or parmesan if tolerated.

Note: Cooked zucchini, celery, carrots, spinach etc. May also be added.

Linguini with Zucchini

Ingredients:

12 oz. linguine (Reserve 1/2 cup cooking water).

1/4 cup olive oil

2 small or 1 large zucchini, sliced or chunked

1-2 cups diced bell pepper (any color)

3 tablespoons chopped herbs (fresh or dried)

2 teaspoons minced garlic

1/3 -1/2 cup grated Parmesan cheese (topping)

Instructions:

Boil linguine until al dente.

Drain, reserving 1/2 cup cooking water.

In a large skillet, heat olive oil for 30 seconds over medium heat. Add zucchini, bell peppers, herbs & garlic.

Cook for 5 minutes. Season with salt & pepper.

In a large bowl, combine linguine, cooking water & other ingredients.

Top with Parmesan. Yum!

IC WHITE BEAN CHICKEN CHILI

Ingredients

1 tablespoon olive oil

1 cup chopped sweet onion (if tolerated)

1 cup chopped celery

2 sweet bell peppers cored and chopped (red, yellow or orange or green if tolerated)

1 pound ground lean chicken or turkey with no preservatives (for vegetarian chili substitute 1 can of beans and 1 cup of corn)

It is also possible to use 2 cups grilled chicken breast or turkey tenderloin instead of ground

1 tablespoon minced garlic

1 tablespoon all-purpose flour

1 teaspoon ground cumin (if tolerated or substitute dried basil)

1 teaspoon dried oregano

2 cups chicken or vegetable broth low-sodium or with no preservatives

2 15 ounce cans white beans drained and rinsed (mash one can of beans for thicker chili)

1/2 cup low-fat sour cream or plain yogurt (if tolerated)

Salt and pepper to taste

Shredded mild cheddar cheese for topping and/or can chopped mild green chilis if tolerated

In a large pot over medium heat warm the oil. Add chopped veggies and sautee for 5 min. Add chicken or turkey and cook through at least 5 minutes. Omit for vegetarian chili.

Add the garlic, flour, cumin (or basil) and oregano. Cook, stirring over low heat 2 minutes. Add the broth while stirring. Increase heat and bring to a boil stirring occasionally. Reduce heat to simmering and cook 10 minutes longer.

Add the beans and simmer another 10 minutes. Mash 1 can of the beans for thicker chili. Add a third can of beans and corn for vegetarian chili.

Stir in sour cream or yogurt. Season with salt and pepper.

Ladle into bowls and top with shredded cheddar and green chilis. May be served over rice, quinoa or other cooked grains. Add a warm piece of corn bread for a more hearty meal. Serves about 6.

Quinoa Salad with Apples – IC friendly side dish

Prep time: a few hours (quinoa needs to cool)

Serves: 6-8

Ingredients:

1 cup quinoa (keen-wa), rinsed

1 tsp olive oil

2 cups water

2 Tbsp honey

2 tsp lemon zest or 1 tsp lemon extract (if tolerated)

½ tsp sea salt

3 Tbsp olive oil

1 medium fuji apple, peeled and diced

1 cup finely chopped celery

1/3 cup finely chopped fresh parsley

½ cup coarsely chopped toasted almonds

1/3 cup organic or untreated raisins, brown or golden (if tolerated)

Instructions:

In a medium-sized saucepan bring quinoa, water and a tsp olive oil to a boil. Reduce heat, cover and simmer 15 minutes until quinoa is tender and water absorbed stirring occasionally to prevent sticking. Remove from heat, transfer to a loosely covered dish and cool.

In a small bowl, whisk together honey, lemon zest or extract and salt. Gradually whisk in olive oil until blended.

Add apple, celery parsley, almonds and raisings to cooled quinoa. Mix well.

Pour dressing over mixture and stir. Serve or refrigerate.

Ideas for substitution or addition:

Exchange walnuts for almonds

Exchange brown raisins for golden

Exchange parsley for mint

a dd spinach or kale

Add coconut shredded or flaked

Upside Down Fruit Pie – IC Friendly!

Ingredients:

1 can blueberry or apple pie filling, as pure of additives as possible (a good brand low in additives is Lucky Leaf brand. Otherwise, create your own pie filling using fresh fruit)

1 15-ounce can pears, drained and diced

1 package Dr. Oetker yellow cake mix

1 cup butter or margarine, melted

1 cup chopped almonds or cashews

Instructions:

Heat oven to 350 degrees. Grease a 9×13-inch baking pan.

Pour pie filling into pan & spread evenly. Arrange diced pears over the filling.

Sprinkle the dry cake mix evenly over the fruit. Drizzle the melted butter over all & covering completely. Top with nuts.

Bake 60 minutes. Let cool 5 minutes, turn upside down on plate. Serve warm with whipped cream and enjoy!

Fruity Gelatin Salad – IC Friendly Dessert

Ingredients:

3 envelopes Knox unflavored gelatin

1/4 cup sugar

2 cups mango juice, heated to boiling (Ceres brand from Meijer's)

2 1/2 cups plain Greek yogurt

1 cup diced or sliced canned pears, drained (reserve syrup)

Use any combination to equal 2 cups: sliced bananas, chopped apples (Gala or Fuji), blueberries, brown raisins, chopped almonds

Instructions:

In a large bowl, mix unflavored gelatin with sugar.

Add hot juice and stir until gelatin is dissolved.

With wire whip or rotary beater, blend in yogurt & reserved syrup.

Chill, stirring occasionally, until mixture resembles unbeaten egg whites. Stir in pears, fruit and nuts.

Pour into 13 x 9 inch pan. Chill until firm. To serve, cut into squares.

Honey Apple Slaw – IC Friendly Salad

This sweet dish gives a good mix of fruit, veggies and protein (Greek yogurt), and serves as a nice salad to make ahead and bring in your lunch to school or work, or to bring as a dish to pass at a gathering.

Makes six one-cup servings.

Ingredients:

5 cups thinly sliced cabbage (Packaged angel hair cabbage works well).

2 cups chopped Fuji apples

1/2 cup pure plain Greek yogurt

3 tablespoons honey (or more to taste)

1/8 teaspoon salt

Instructions:

Combine cabbage and apples in large bowl.

Combine remaining ingredients in small bowl; stir or whisk well.

Add small bowel mixture to cabbage mixture, tossing to coat.

Cover & chill.

Variations:

To add a little crunch, you can add a nut of your choice — almonds or walnuts work well and are IC friendly.

Sliced or shredded radish and/or carrots may add some color as well.

Raisins can add some sweetness.

Try adding shredded or chopped fresh fennel; or replacing cabbage all together with fennel.

California Crunch Salad – IC Friendly Side Dish

Here's a tasty green salad for the holidays.

Ingredients:

1 16-ounce bag broccoli slaw

2 bunches green onions, chopped (if tolerated)

1/2 cup slivered almonds

2 tablespoons butter or margarine

1 package Ramen noodles, dry, uncooked, and crushed (discard seasoning packet)

1/4 cup sunflower seeds

Dressing

1/2 cup vegetable or olive oil

4 tablespoons sugar

4 tablespoons honey

Salt & pepper, if desired

Instructions:

Melt butter in fry pan, stir in almonds and crushed Ramen noodles.

Lightly brown and cool on paper towel.

Mix broccoli slaw and green onions in bowl.

Add almond and noodle mixture with desired amount of dressing just before serving.

Enjoy!

Rich Rice with Mushrooms and Spinach – IC Friendly Side Dish

Makes 6 servings

Ingredients:

4 cups cooked brown rice, divided

2 tablespoons butter or margarine

1 sweet onion, chopped

8 ounces fresh mushrooms, sliced

1 cup pure sour cream

1 cup finely chopped spinach (packed) May use fresh or well-drained frozen spinach

1 cup grated Swiss or cheddar cheese

Salt and pepper to taste

Instructions:

Spoon half the rice into shallow 2-quart greased baking dish. Melt butter in large skillet. Add onion, mushrooms and seasonings. Cook over medium heat until onions are soft but not brown. Remove from heat; stir in sour cream. Spread mixture over rice. Cover with spinach. Top with remaining rice; sprinkle with cheese. Bake at 350 degrees for 30-35 minutes.

IC Friendly Black Bean and Butternut Squash Burritos

Yield: 4 burritos or 3.5 cups of filling

Ingredients:

1 medium butternut squash, peeled, cubed, and roasted

*You can also try substituting butternut squash for sweet potato or pumpkin.

1/2 cup uncooked short grain brown rice (yields: 1.5 cups cooked)

1-2 tsp olive oil

1 cup chopped sweet onion, if tolerated

2 garlic cloves, minced

1 sweet red bell pepper, chopped

1 tsp kosher salt, or to taste

2 tsp ground cumin, or to taste, if tolerated

One 15-oz can black beans (about 1.5-2 cups cooked), drained and rinsed

3/4 cup mild cheddar cheese

4 tortilla wraps (large or x-large)

Toppings of choice: (avocado, sour cream, spinach/lettuce, etc)

Directions:

1. Preheat oven to 425 degrees F and line a large glass dish with tinfoil. Drizzle olive oil on squash and give a shake of salt and

pepper. Coat with hands. Roast chopped butternut squash for 45 mins. or until tender.

2. Cook brown rice (for directions, see here)

3. In a large skillet over medium-low heat, add oil, onion, and minced garlic. Sautee for about 5 minutes, stirring frequently. Now add in salt and seasonings and stir well.

4. Add chopped sweet red bell pepper, black beans, and cooked rice and sauté for another 10 mins. On low.

5. When butternut squash is tender remove from oven and cool slightly. Add 1.5 cups of the cooked butternut squash to the skillet and stir well. You can mash the squash with a fork if some pieces are too large. Add cheddar cheese and heat another couple minutes.

6. Add bean filling to tortilla along with desired toppings. Wrap and serve. Leftover filling can be reheated the next day for lunch in a wrap or as a salad topper.

Red Lentil and Squash Stew

Yield: about 4 servings

Ingredients:

1 tsp Extra virgin olive oil

1 sweet onion, chopped (if tolerated)

3 garlic cloves, minced

1 tbsp turmeric (if tolerated), or more to taste

1 carton broth (4 cups)

1 cup red lentils

3 cups cooked butternut squash

1 cup greens of choice

Fresh grated ginger, to taste (optional)

Kosher salt & black pepper, to taste (I used about 1/2 tsp salt)

Instructions:

1. In a large pot, add olive oil and chopped onion and minced garlic. Saute for about 5 minutes over low-medium heat.

2. Stir in turmeric and cook another couple minutes. Add broth and lentils and bring to a boil. Reduce heat and cook for 10 minutes.

3. Stir in cooked butternut squash and greens of choice. Cook over medium heat for about 5-8 minutes. Season with salt, pepper, and add some freshly grated ginger to taste.

Fruity Gelatin Salad – IC Friendly Dessert

Ingredients:

3 envelopes Knox unflavored gelatin

1/4 cup sugar

2 cups mango juice, heated to boiling (Ceres brand from Meijer's)

2 1/2 cups plain Greek yogurt

1 cup diced or sliced canned pears, drained (reserve syrup)

Use any combination to equal 2 cups: sliced bananas, chopped apples (Gala or Fuji), blueberries, brown raisins, chopped almonds

Instructions:

In a large bowl, mix unflavored gelatin with sugar.

Add hot juice and stir until gelatin is dissolved.

With wire whip or rotary beater, blend in yogurt & reserved syrup.

Chill, stirring occasionally, until mixture resembles unbeaten egg whites. Stir in pears, fruit and nuts.

Pour into 13 x 9 inch pan. Chill until firm. To serve, cut into squares.

C Friendly Fruit Gelatin

Let's keep it simple this week with a gelatin recipe.

Ingredients:

1/4 cup cold water

1/2 cup boiling water

1 1/4 cups fruit juice (Ceres brand Mango juice is made of pure pear and mango juice, and is available at Meijer stores)

1 packet Knox gelatin

3 tablespoons honey

1 can pear or mango slices, drained (Note: The drained juice may be used for part of the fruit juice measure above)

Instructions:

Soften gelatin by soaking in cold water for a few minutes.

Dissolve in boiling water. Add honey.

When cool add fruit juice and drained fruit.

Variation: One cup of cottage cheese may be added with the fruit.

IC Friendly Good Morning Granola

It's been a while, let's do breakfast this week!

Ingredients:

3 cups old-fashioned rolled oats

1 cup sliced almonds

1/2 cup (no additives) shredded sweetened coconut

2 tablespoons wheat germ

1/2 teaspoon salt

1/2 teaspoon ground cinnamon (if tolerated)

2 tablespoons pure vegetable oil

1/2 cup pure maple syrup

2 tablespoons firmly packed brown sugar

1 cup brown raisins (if tolerated). Add or substitute dried blueberries, dried apples or dried apricots (if tolerated).

Directions:

Heat oven to 350 degrees.

Combine oats almonds, coconut, wheat germ, salt & cinnamon in large bowl.

Combine oil, syrup & brown sugar in another bowl & pour over oat mixture.

Toss until well coated.

Spread evenly in 13 x 9-inch pan.

Bake 30 minutes or until golden brown, stirring frequently. Cool completely. Stir in raisins or other tolerated dried fruits.

Store in airtight container at room temperature.

Makes 5 cups.

IC friendly Quick Oats Granola

Ingredients

3 cups quick oats

1/3 cup brown sugar

1/3 cup honey

1 teaspoon olive oil

1 teaspoon water

Salt to taste

1/4 teaspoon vanilla extract (up to a teaspoon if you prefer)

1/4 cup peanut butter (optional or try almond butter)

1/4 teaspoon cinnamon if tolerated

Instructions

Mix together all ingredients in a large bowl adding more water if needed to ensure it is mixed thoroughly. Spread on a large cookie sheet with an edge.

Bake at 250 degrees for 1 hour to 1.5 hours until crisp and golden stirring and checking every 20 min. After cooling add 1-2 cups toasted almonds and/or coconut if desired.

This is a nice addition to top your morning yogurt along with fresh or frozen blueberries.

Add dried instead of fresh blueberries and enjoy with milk or just like it is!

IC Friendly Blueberry Smoothie

If you are skipping breakfast, aside from dragging in the morning, you may be missing some essential nutrients. Here's an idea so you don't derail your New Year's Resolution to eat more healthy: A smoothie recipe that's good for you, tastes delish and keeps your bladder happy. But remember, a dietitian's taste buds may be a little more sugar sensitive, so feel free to add another teaspoon or so of honey if it isn't sweet enough for you. Don't worry, honey is only 20 calories per teaspoon.

BLUEBERRY BLAST

Yields: 2 servings

Ingredients

1 cup lowfat milk or almond milk (8 grams protein in a cup of milk, 1 gram protein in a cup of almond milk)

1/2 cup Greek style plain yogurt

1/2 tsp vanilla extract

2 teaspoons honey to taste (optional if using vanilla yogurt or sweetened almond milk)

1 cup baby spinach or kale, stems removed, washed, dried and chopped

1 cup fresh or frozen blueberries or if you tolerate bananas: 1/2 cup blueberries and 1/2 ripe banana, sliced

1/4 cup quick cooking oats (you can use old fashioned, just may need to blend longer)

1/4 avocado (optional) added if you don't tolerate or like bananas

Instructions

Place 1/2 of all ingredients into a blender. Cover and blend a minute until creamy and smooth. Repeat for the second serving. Serve immediately in a 16 oz glass or freeze in a freezer safe container with a lid and leave 1 inch of space for expansion. Or cover and refrigerate for the next day.

Growing teens and athletes can add nut butter and whey protein powder (may be IC safe for some). If you want to avoid the vitamin C in protein powders that can be an IC irritant, but you want extra protein, dry, non-fat milk powder adds 3 grams protein and 25 calories per tablespoon. Garnish with fresh mint leaf or coconut if desired.

Roughly: 200 calories, 30 grams carb and 18 grams protein per 1/2 recipe

Peanut Butter Banana Oat Breakfast Cookies – IC Friendly!

This recipe has been adapted slightly to be ic friendly. It is a great option for an on-the-go healthy breakfast or a quick afternoon snack!

Ingredients

2 bananas, mashed until smooth & creamy

1/3 cup peanut butter – creamy or chunky

2/3 cup unsweetened applesauce

1 scoop whey-based protein powder (optional** can be made without, cookie will just be lower in protein)

1 tsp vanilla extract

1 1/2 cups quick oatmeal – uncooked (or use old fashioned oats for more oatmeal texture)

1/4 cup chopped nuts (peanut, walnut, or your favorite)

1/4 cup carob, white chocolate, peanut butter, butterscotch or high-quality dark chocolate chips (**optional — based on ic tolerance)

Instructions:

Preheat heat oven to 350 degrees.

In a large bowl, mix mashed banana & peanut butter until completely combined then add in the applesauce, vanilla protein powder & the extract(s) ~ mix again until all are completely combined.

Add in the oatmeal & nuts to the banana mixture & combine. (** add the optional carob / chocolate chips at this time if you want them mixed throughout)

Let dough rest for 10 minutes.

Drop cookie dough, by spoonfuls, onto a parchment paper lined cookie sheet & flatten cookies into rounds. (** if you just want the carob / chocolate chips on the top of the cookies, add now)

Bake cookies approx. 30 minutes, or until golden brown & done. Remove from oven & let rest on cookie sheet for 5 minutes, then move to cooling rack. (if you want the traditional fork tong marks on the cookies, use a pizza cutter or sharp knife to score the tops of the cookies while they're still warm)

When cookies are completely cool, store in a covered container. Enjoy!

No-Bake Fudge Nut Balls – Quick and Easy IC Friendly Holiday Cookies

It's time to think CHRISTMAS COOKIES! Here's a quick and easy, IC Friendly recipe many of your family and friends will enjoy just as much as you will. See if they can even tell its not made with chocolate or cocoa!

Ingredients:

1/2 cup butter or margarine

2 cups granulated sugar

1/2 cup milk

1/2 cup carob powder (Chatfield's brand available at Harvest Health stores in West Michigan, or here at Amazon.com online)

1 teaspoon vanilla or almond extract

2 cups oatmeal (not instant)

1/2 cup finely ground almonds

Instructions:

Combine butter, sugar and milk in saucepan. Let mixture come to a boil over medium heat, and simmer 3 minutes. Remove from heat.

Into saucepan mixture, whisk carob powder, then vanilla.

In separate bowl, place oats and 1/2 cup finely ground nuts.

Add saucepan mixture to bowl with oats and nuts. Mix thoroughly, set aside until warm.

Form into balls about the the size of a quarter in diameter. Roll in granulated sugar.

Note: If dough becomes too cool and turns crumbly, place bowl in microwave to re-warm.

IC Texas Sheet Cake

Carob is an alternative to chocolate. Use it in powder or chip form for baking and try things you wouldn't normally be able to eat... like this wonderful Texas Sheet Cake recips that is IC diet friendly!

Ingredients

2 sticks (one cup) butter or margarine

1 cup water

4 tablespoons carob powder (Chatfield's brand is sold at Harvest Health stores in West Michigan)

1/4 teaspoon salt

Place above ingredients into a medium saucepan; bring to a boil; remove from heat & add:

2 cups flour

2 cups sugar 2 teaspoons baking soda

1 cup pure Greek yogurt (Oikos plain works well)

1 egg

Instructions

Mix all & pour into greased cookie sheet WITH EDGE. Place into 350 degree oven for 20 minutes.

Using the same unwashed saucepan add:

1/2 cup butter or margarine

1/3 cup milk

4 tablespoons carob powder

Bring to boil; remove from heat & add 1 teaspoon pure vanilla, 1 cup chopped nuts & 1 pound powdered sugar. Leave mixture on stove & frost cake with the mixture 15 minutes after the cake comes out of the oven.

Homemade Breakfast Bars – IC Friendly

Ingredients:

1/3 c honey

1/2 c almond or peanut butter

1 tsp vanilla extract

1 1/4 c gluten free crispy rice cereal

1 c gluten free uncooked oats

2 Tbsp ground flax seed if tolerated or ground almonds

2 1/2 tsp unsweetened carob powder (optional available at health food stores or online)

Optional: Add your favorite tolerated dried fruit — blueberries, golden or regular raisins, pear or apple chunks.

Instructions:

Microwave honey and nut butter 30-45 sec or until bubbly in a glass bowl. Add vanilla.

Combine rice cereal, oats, flax seed or almonds and carob powder in a large bowl. Stir in honey nut butter mixture until well combined with a spatula as is very sticky.

Pour into lined 8×8 pan and press down until level. Cool then cover and put in refrigerator at least 30 minutes.

Cut into bars with sharp knife sprayed with cooking spray. Cut into 8 or more bars, wrap in plastic wrap and refrigerate. Leave out 5 min and enjoy!

CONCLUSION

The nutrients in foods help strengthen your immune system, heal wounds, stimulate nerve transmission, keep your blood flowing normally, and promote overall health. A balanced diet with a wide variety of items from all food groups is the best diet for interstitial cystitis (IC). It is also the best diet for everyone. The only the difference is that those with IC should limit some foods and beverages.

Restricting too many foods and beverages can affect your well-being in a bad way. So it is very important to replace the nutrients provided by bothersome foods and beverages with alternative options. Fortunately, it's easy to find foods and beverages that substitute for the ones that must be restricted to help manage bladder symptoms.

To get the nutrition you need:

Aim for a variety of foods.

Eat in moderation—often restaurants serve larger portions than you will need. So, ask for a doggie bag!

Drink adequate fluids—pee and then peek, your urine should be a pale yellow color.

Watch you intake of sugar, salt, alcohol, and fat (specifically saturated fat, trans fats, and cholesterol from animal and processed products). These recommendations hold true for everyone.

Check the Nutrition Facts label and ingredient lists for the amounts of saturated fat, sodium, and added sugars in the foods and beverages you choose, as well as for your IC trigger items.

Made in United States
Troutdale, OR
02/09/2025

28724772R00056